<u>Juice Recipes</u>

Delicious Fruit and Vegetable Juices

By: Kevin Kerr

In no way is it legal to reproduce, duplicate, or transmit any part of this document in either electronic means or in printed format. Recording of this publication is strictly prohibited and any storage of this document is not allowed unless with written permission from the publisher.

Table of Contents

Introduction

There are three types of juicers that one has to choose from which include manual devices which work well for citrus fruits and wheatgrass, centrifugal, and masticating which are both electrical. Centrifugal juicers use a spinning grater-like blade to extract the nutrition from fruits and vegetables and work well for carrots and beets. Masticating juicers are a little more money than centrifugal but well worth it because they produce a fresh-pressed juice that preserves all the enzymes and vitamins. If you want to juice greens, which is probably one of healthiest vegetables one can consume, this is the juicer for you. It is an easy way to incorporate more raw foods into your diet. Raw food is anything that isn't heated over 118 degrees so that the precious enzymes aren't destroyed. Juices are so fantastic for your health because they don't require any energy to break down the food providing your with quick, long lasting energy that won't make you crash. In order for food to digest it must be metabolized and broken down by enzymes. Science has recently discovered that our bodies can only produce so many enzymes in this lifetime which is the number one reason to eat as much raw food as you enjoy.

For all recipes I recommended using local organic produce as much as possible due to the harmful chemicals that are used when growing conventional produce. However, this is not always possible so here is a list of fruits and vegetables with the typical lowest pesticide contents: asparagus avocados, bananas, broccoli, carrots, cabbage, eggplant, grapefruits, kiwi, mangoes, mushrooms, pineapple, romaine lettuce, sweet peas, sweet potatoes, and watermelon. I highly recommend that all other produce you consume should be organically grown or wild harvested such as dandelion greens.

You need an electrical powered juicer to complete nearly all of the recipes in this book. I got mine my first one for five dollars at the Salvation Army, my second one for three dollars at a yard sale, my third one for free on the side of the road for free and my fourth one at the Salvation Army. Juicing is simple, delicious, and possibly one of the best activities you could be doing a daily basis for your physical health. A fresh juice is a great breakfast to allow digestion to catch up from the previous day, which helps with nutrient assimilation. It separates the nutrients and water from the fiber which gives your body a rest from having to break down food thus allowing it to use more of it's energy towards healing and doing the things you love. All juices listed here serve 1 to 3 people. The following tips will help you get started:

- lemon in your juice acts as a natural preservative that will keep in fresh in the refrigerator for several days

- if possible drink your juice right after making it to receive the highest nutritional content
- have a little fat such as avocado, olive oil, coconut oil, nuts or seeds with your juice to increase nutrient absorption
- always turn on machine before putting in your produce
- bananas and avocados aren't the best choice for juicing
- apples and carrots pair well with the bitter taste of certain vegetables
- juices are a fantastic caffeine and/or meal replacement
- if the produce is organic juice all of it including beet greens and lemon peels
- for a thicker juice add back in some of the fiber
- when juicing greens it helps to roll them up or juice them with a firmer vegetable such as carrots to get the most juice from them
- mixing juice with superfoods or fresh whole fruits such as bananas in a blender is a great way to create a delicious smoothie
- you can save leftover pulp and add it to salads or other healthy meals you create
- freeze fresh juice in popsicle molds for healthy frozen treats

10 Juice Recipes

Sweet Surrender
- 1 pineapple
- 7 gala apples
- 7 blood blood red oranges
- 1 lemon
- 3 stalks swiss chard

Healer
- 4 stalks celery
- 1 small beet (including greens)
- 1 pound lacinto kale
- ½ pound carrots
- 1 red delicious apple

Deep Green
- 3 cups spinach
- 4 stalks celery
- 2 leaves swiss chard
- 2 stalks broccoli
- 1 golden delicious apple
- 1 bartlett pear
- thumb-sized chunk of ginger root

Summertime Heaven
- ¾ parts watermelon(s)
- ¼ part pear(s)

Skin Healer
- 3 grapefruits
- 2 mangoes
- ½ beet
- ½ lemon

Liver Detox
- 3 beets
- 4 oranges

Nourisher
- 2 leaves swiss chard
- 2 cups strawberries
- 1 apple of choice
- 1 medium-sized cucumber

Green Powerhouse

- 4 stalks celery
- 4 stalks kale
- 3 leaves romaine lettuce
- 1 medium-sized cucumber
- 10-20 mint leaves
- ginger root
- ½ lemon (peel and all if organic)

Refreshing Cleanse

- 5 stalks celery
- 2 cups grapes

Simple Treat

- 2 pounds carrots
- 2 inch slice of a fresh whole pineapple

Juiced Love
- 7 stalks kale
- 2 cups strawberries
- 1 medium-sized apple
- 1 medium-sized cucumber

Carrot Beet Fast
- 5 pounds carrots
- 1 beet
- 3 teaspoons organic maca powder
- 2 teaspoons ceylon cinnamon powder

Juice vegetables, then stir or shake in the maca and cinnamon. The results yield a delicious drink that will satisfy your body all day!

Sweet Greens
- 4 cups spinach
- 1 apple
- 2 large carrots

Sweet Celery Juice

- 10 stalks celery
- 2 pears
- ginger root

Red Heaven

- 1 beet
- 2 sticks rhubarb
- 1 red bell pepper
- 1 apple
- 1 pear
- 2 carrots
- ginger root

The Usual

- 3 pounds of carrots
- 1 beetroot
- ½ of a Lemon

Summertime Delight

- 4 pounds of watermelon
- 2 pears
- 1 whole lime
- 1 peach

Green Dream

- 10 leaves of your favorite kale
- 4 stalks of celery
- 1 whole cucumber
- 2 of your favorite organic apples
- 10 stalks of cilantro
- A handful of blueberries
- A handful of blackberries

Breakfast and Lunch

- 1 grapefruit
- 15 cranberries
- 2 oranges
- ½ of a mango
- 1 inch slice of a fresh pineapple

Woah

- 3 handfuls of Strawberries
- 2 handfuls of Red Raspberries
- 1 persimmon
- 2 asian ears
- 50 concord grapes (about 4 to five cups)
- 2 bunches

Juiced Love

- 4 kiwis
- 5 peaches
- 1 lime
- 6 stalks of rainbow swiss chard
- 1 cucumber

Chlorophyll Central

- 1 pound of spinach
- 10 stalks of kale
- 1 cucumber
- 3 stalks of celery
- 8 kiwis

Passionate Pomegranate

- 3 pomegranates (Seed and all) (Not the shell or white flesh inside)
- 4 passion fruits
- 1 head of romaine Lettuce
- 1 beetroot
- 1 lemon

Longevity in a Cup

- 15 carrots
- 1 beetroot
- ½ of a lemon
- 10 cranberries
- 1 whole head and stalk of broccoli
- 5 leaves of kale

Natural Tang

- 10 carrots
- 7 oranges
- 2 mangos
- 5 peaches
- sliver of a habanero pepper
- 1 inch chunk of ginger root

Skin Lover

- 1 pound of carrots
- 1 large cucumber
- 2 stalks celery

Tropical Delight

- 1 guava
- 1 papaya
- 1 pineapple
- 1 orange
- 1 mango

Magnificent Melon

- ½ of a cantaloupe
- 3 carrots
- 1 apple
- 1 orange
- 1 grapefruit

Cucumber Carrot

- 1 pound of carrots
- 2 cucumbers

Real Good Morning

- 2 or 3 carrots
- 1 apple
- ½ of a beet
- 1 pint of strawberries

Sensational Start

- ½ of a pineapple
- 1 orange
- 1 cup of strawberries
- 1 bunch of red grapes
- 1 bunch of parsley

Pineapple Delight

- 1 whole pineapple
- 2 oranges
- 1 bunch of cilantro
- 1 bunch of mint

Lemon Ginger Elixir

- 1 lemon
- 1 thumb-sized chunk of ginger
- 8 ounces of spinach
- 2 apples
- 1 bunch of parsley
- 1 bunch of cilantro
- 1 cucumber

Liver Cleanser

- 1 apple
- 1 beet
- 1 pound of carrots
- 2 lemons
- 2 pears

Lemelon

- 4 cups watermelon
- 1 cucumber
- 1 lemon
- 1 lime

Cucumber Cleanse

- 2 or 3 cucumbers
- 1 pound of carrots
- 1 apple
- 1 grapefruit

Mint Melon

- 1 bunch of mint
- 1 stalk of celery
- 1 cucumber

Berry Blast

- 1 cup blackberries
- 1 cup strawberries
- 1 cup raspberries
- 1 cup blueberries
- 1 head of your favorite greens
- 3 cups watermelon

Carrot Turmeric Apple
- 1 pound of carrots
- 2 apples
- 1 thumb-sized of turmeric

Mango Love
- 1 mango
- 3 kiwis
- 2 or 3 carrots

Early Morning
- ½ pineapple
- 1 mango
- 1 tomato
- 3 stalks swiss chard
- ½ lemon
- 1 sweet potato
- 3 stalks celery

Hawaiian Treat
- 1 papaya
- 1 guava
- 1 pineapple
- 1 pound of rambutans
- 1 pound of lychee

Perfect Papaya
- 1 papaya
- 1 pineapple

Melonator
- ½ cantaloupe
- ½ cantaloupe
- ½ watermelon
- 2 cucumbers

Perfect Sunrise
- ½ pineapple
- 2 mangoes

Peachy Pear
- 3 peaches
- 2 pears

Detoxer
- ½ pineapple
- 1 orange
- 1 papaya
- 1 mango
- 2 or 3 carrots
- ½ lime
- ½ lemon
- 1 bunch of your favorite greens

Beelieve It
- 1 beet
- 3 or 4 carrots
- 2 oranges
- 1 cucumber

Green Carrot
- 2 pounds of carrots
- 2 bunches of parsley

Rainbow Morning

- ½ cucumber
- 1 yellow bell pepper
- 1 tomato
- 1 orange
- 4 ounces of spinach
- 3 stalks celery
- 2 or 3 carrots

Blueberry Grapple

- 1 lemon
- 1 cup blueberries
- 1 cup red grapes
- 1 apple

Mexican Juice

- 1 large red bell pepper
- 2 stalks of celery
- ½ lime
- 6 stalks of cilantro
- 1 apple

Spicy Tomato

- 1 tomato
- 3 carrots
- 2 stalks of celery
- 1 thumb-sized chunk of ginger
- 1 thumb-sized or horseradish root
- 5 stalks of cilantro
- 2 radishes
- 1 clove of garlic

Pearfect Grape Juice

- 3 pears
- 2 cups of your favorite grapes

Pineapple Punch

- 2 cups of pineapple
- 1 pint of strawberries
- 1 mango

Crazy Cantaloupe

- 1 cantaloupe
- 3 pears

Stress Reducer

- 4 stalks celery
- ½ fennel bulb
- ½ head of romaine lettuce
- ½ pineapple

Perfect Peppermint

- 1 cup of peppermint leaves
- 3 oranges
- 3 apples

Apple Ginger Juice

- 5 apples
- 1 lemon
- 1 thumb-sized chunk of ginger

Skin Lover

- 1 cucumber
- 1 bunch of parsley
- 1 apple
- 3 or 4 carrots

Red Glory
- 1 beet
- 1 tomato
- 1 red bell pepper
- 1 cucumber
- ½ pound of carrots
- 3 leaves of red cabbage

Natural Punch
- 3 cups kale
- 2 cups parsley
- 2 cups spinach
- 1 apple
- 4 stalks celery
- 1 orange bell pepper

Paradise
- 1 papaya
- 2 oranges
- ½ pineapple
- 1 lime
- 1 thumb-sized chunk of ginger

Islander

- 1 pineapple
- 1 pint strawberries
- 2 apples
- 1 papaya

Melon Ginger

- 1 thumb-sized chunk of ginger
- 1/2 cantaloupe
- 1 pint strawberries
- 1 orange

Crafty Cabbage

- 1 thumb-sized chunk of ginger
- 2 stalks celery
- 5 leaves of cabbage
- 1 yellow bell pepper
- 1 pear

Quick Breakfast

- 1 cantaloupe
- ½ pound of carrots
- ½ lemon
- 1 apple

Fat Buster

- 4 carrots
- 3 stalks celery
- 1 cucumber
- 1 small bunch of cilantro
- 1 beet
- 1 apple

Kiwi Passion

- 1 passion fruit
- 1 cup grapes
- 2 kiwis

Cranberry Pear Juice

- 3 pears
- 1 peach
- 2 cups cranberries
- ½ pineapple

Ravishing Red Raspberry

- 2 pints red raspberries
- 2 oranges
- 1 lime

Fabulous Forager
- 1 head purple cabbage
- 2 cups red grapes
- 2 cups blueberries
- 4 stalks kale

A Taste of the Forrest
- 1 bunch of cilantro
- 1 bunch of parsley
- 5 stalks of kale
- 1 beet
- 1 cucumber
- 1 lemon
- 1 thumb-sized chunk of turmeric
- 1 thumb-sized chunk of ginger

Revitalizer
- 3 apples
- 3 stalks celery
- 1 cucumber
- 1 lime
- 1 thumb-sized chunk of ginger

Lonely Veggie

- 3 oranges
- 1 apple
- 1 pear
- 1 cucumber
- 1 zucchini

Green Delight

- 5 stalks kale
- 5 stalks swiss chard
- 1 cucumber
- 1 apple
- 1 orange
- 7 clementines

Citrus Twist

- 1 cucumber
- 1 lemon
- 1 lime
- 3 kiwis
- 2 apples
- 1 thumb-sized chunk of turmeric

Berry Pearific

- 4 pears
- 3 cups watermelon
- 1 pint black raspberries

The Melon Musketeers

- 3 cups watermelon
- 3 cups honeydew
- 3 cups cantaloupe
- 1 cucumber

Summer Treat

- 1 pint strawberries
- ½ pineapple
- 3 cups red grapes

Berry Good Treat

- 1 cup cranberries
- 1 cup strawberries
- 1 cup raspberries
- 1 cup blueberries
- add to 1 cup of filtered or spring water

The Motivator

- 4 stalks of celery
- 1 cucumber
- 4 ounces of spinach
- 1 apple
- 1 orange bell pepper

Kool Kiwi

- 3 kiwi fruits
- ½ pineapple
- 1 orange
- 1 thumb-sized chunk of turmeric

Peachy Apricot

- 2 peaches
- 2 apricots
- 1 pear
- 1 apple

Spicy Orange
- 1 thumb-sized chunk of ginger
- 3 oranges
- ½ honeydew
- ½ lime

Perfection
- 1 tomato
- ½ red leaf lettuce
- 3 stalks celery
- 1 carrot
- 1 yellow red bell pepper

Tangy Berry
- 1 pint strawberries
- 1 pint red raspberries
- 1 lemon
- 1 pound of spinach

Cranberry Apple Juice
- 1 pint of strawberries
- 1 apples

Love Elixir

- 1 peach
- 2 cups of red grapes
- 2 cups of strawberries
- 1 apple

Ravishing Rainbow

- 3 stalks celery
- 3 carrots
- 1 cucumber
- 1 yellow squash
- 1 apple

Ultimate Vegetable Juice

- 2 carrots
- 2 stalks celery
- 1/2 beet
- 1 small bunch of parsley
- ½ head of lettuce
- 1 small bunch of watercress
- 2 ounces of spinach
- 3 tomatoes
- sea salt to taste

Tropical Love

- 1 orange
- 1 pineapple
- 1 mango
- 1 papaya
- 1 guava

Papple Pear

- 2 apples
- 2 pears
- ½ pineapple

Body Lover

- 2 cups grapes
- 2 large oranges
- 2 lemons

Citrusy Grape

- 2 cups of grapes
- 3 oranges
- 1 lemon

Ginger Melon

- 1 thumb-sized chunk of ginger
- 3 cups watermelon
- 3 cups cantaloupe

Green Heaven

- 4 ounces of spinach
- 1 head of broccoli
- 3 apples
- 1 lemon

Fast Morning

- 3 apples
- 3 pears
- 3 oranges

Apple Pie

- 4 cups butternut squash
- 3 apples
- 1 teaspoon of cinnamon powder

V5

- 3 tomatoes
- 5 leaves of cabbage
- 1 bunch of parsley
- 3 stalks of celery
- 1 cucumber
- 1 thumb-sized chunk of turmeric
- salt and pepper to taste

Sweet Intention

- 1 sweet potato
- 3 carrots
- 1 beet
- 1 bell pepper
- 1 pear
- 1 apple
- 1 orange
- ½ head of bok choy